Angioedema

A Comprehensive Beginners Guide To Angioedema Diagnosis And Treatment

Dr. Kelly Rowland

Table of Contents

Chapter One

Angioedema

Hives are raised, purple dots or welts that seem at the pores and skin. These welts frequently itch. The scientific time period for hives is urticaria. Angioedema is swollen tissues below the pores and skin. The situations frequently arise collectively as a part of a hypersensitive reaction.

What are hives (urticaria)?

Hives are raised purple bumps (welts) or splotches at the pores and skin. They are a form of swelling at the floor of your pores and skin. They show up whilst your frame has a hypersensitive reaction to an allergen, a substance that's innocent to maximum human beings. But also, can arise in autoimmune situations or systemic situations, if hives closing for an extended duration of time.

Hives can be itchy, or you may experience them burning or stinging. They may be as small as a pinprick or as large as a dinner plate. The scientific call for hives is urticaria.

Sometimes, the welts from hives be part of collectively to shape large regions referred to as plaques. Hives have a tendency to vanish inside 24 hours, even though they'll be substantive for numerous days or longer.

What is swelling (angioedema)?

Angioedema is a sort of swelling that may be associated with hives, however may be a remoted event. It most usually reasons swelling in deep layers of tissue across the eyes, lips and face. Your hands, toes, throat, intestines and genitals may swell.

People who get hives may also get angioedema on the equal time. Sometimes human beings have angioedema without hives.

Swelling from angioedema may be itchy, and may every so often be painful. It generally is going away in an afternoon or. In intense situations, your throat, airway and digestive tract may swell. These reactions may be life-threatening.

How not are hives and angioedema?

About 20% of human beings will expand hives at the least as soon as. Angioedema through itself takes place much less frequently.

Who's maximum in all likelihood to get hives (urticaria) or angioedema?

Anyone can get hives or angioedema. Hives are extra not than angioedema. People who react to many distinctive forms of allergens may also get hives frequently. Some human beings get hives simply as soon as or only some instances of their lives.

What are the forms of hives (urticaria) and angioedema?

There are distinctive forms of hives (urticaria) and angioedema, along with:

Acute: Hives or swelling that closing for much less than six weeks are taken into consideration acute, that means they arrive on suddenly. Allergic reactions to sure meals or medicines frequently reason acute hives and swelling.

Chronic: When hives linger for extra than six weeks, the situation is continual. In 95% of continual situations, no person is aware of what reasons them, though it's miles concept to be autoimmune in nature.

Physical: Some human beings expand hives and swelling in particular situations. Hives may pop up whilst you're withinside the bloodless, warmth or sun. Some human beings react to vibrations or strain, or workout and sweating. Physical hives generally seem inside an hour after publicity.

There are 4 essential types of angioedema: Allergic, idiopathic, drug-brought on, and hereditary.

Allergic angioedema

This is the maximum not kind, and it generally impacts people with an allergic reaction to a form of food, a medicine, venom, pollen, or animal dander.

In critical instances, there can be an excessive hypersensitive reaction called anaphylaxis. The throat may also swell, making it difficult for the affected person to breath. Blood strain may also fall suddenly. This is a scientific emergency.

This form of angioedema isn't continual, or long-time period. As quickly because the man or woman identifies which object is inflicting the hypersensitive reaction, they could keep away from it.

Chapter Two

Drug-Brought On Angioedema

Certain medicines can reason angioedema. These consist of angiotensin-changing enzyme

(ACE) inhibitors, a remedy for hypertension, or excessive blood strain.

According to the Merck Manuals, 30 percentage of instances of angioedema which are visible withinside the emergency branch is connected to using ACE inhibitors.

If angioedema stems from the usage of an ACE inhibitor, a healthcare company can prescribe a distinctive form of blood strain medicine.

Another not form of medicine that could reason angioedema is the non-steroidal anti-inflammatory elegance of drugs (NSAIDS) along with ibuprofen or aspirin. These are not painkillers.

Idiopathic angioedema

If a sickness is idiopathic, the reason is unclear. In this case, the physician won't be capable of become aware of a particular reason for angioedema after searching in any respect of the standard reasons.

Hereditary angioedema

Some forms of angioedema are inherited. This manner that numerous human beings withinside the own circle of relatives may also have signs.

Acute episodes of hereditary angioedema do now no longer reply to adrenaline, antihistamine and corticosteroids. Most acute episodes of Type I and II hereditary angioedema aren't life-threatening.

The mainstay of emergency scientific remedy is intravenous C1 inhibitor listen (a blood product).

If that is unavailable, sparkling frozen plasma may be infused, however this every now and then exacerbates the angioedema.

Icatibant, an artificial peptidomimetic drug and bradykinin B2 receptor antagonist, may be utilized in emergencies for the symptomatic remedy of acute assaults of hereditary angioedema in adults with C1-esterase-inhibitor deficiency. It became accredited through the FDA in 2011. In New Zealand, it's miles to be had for domestic use on Special Authority application.

Celanide is a powerful and selective human plasma kallikrein inhibitor this is additionally indicated for the symptomatic remedy of hereditary angioedema, accredited to be used through the FDA in 2009. It is a protease this is answerable for freeing bradykinin from its precursor kininogen. Ecallantide has been suggested to reason anaphylaxis in four% of instances and for this reason has a black container caution withinside the USA.

The risk of an assault may be decreased with the subsequent medicines:

C1 inhibitor listen infused an hour earlier than a surgical procedure

Anabolic steroids (stanazolol, oxandrolone and danazol) to boom circulating degrees of everyday purposeful C1 inhibitor. These have 'male-like' hormonal activity, so may also reason weight gain, menstrual irregularities and virilism.

Tranexamic acid has been utilized in pre-pubertal youngsters and can be powerful in Type III hereditary angioedema.

A monoclonal antibody, lanadelumab, which inhibits energetic plasma kallikrein, has been accredited withinside the USA for the prevention of hereditary angioedema assaults.

What reasons hives (urticaria) and swelling (angioedema)?

Allergens can reason those reactions. An allergen is a substance your frame doesn't like, and your frame's immune machine reacts through liberating chemical compounds referred to as histamines. Histamines are a chemical made through allergic reaction cells (mast cell) and different immune cells (eosinophils, basophils, etc) that is going into overdrive to dispose of the allergen. But your frame may also reply to the flood of histamines through having a hypersensitive reaction that reasons hives and swelling.

People get hives and angioedema from all types of things, along with:

Airborne allergens like tree and grass pollen, mould spores and puppy dander.

Bacterial infections, along with strep throat and urinary tract infections.

Food hypersensitive reactions to milk, peanuts and tree nuts, eggs, fish and shellfish.

Insect stings.

Medication hypersensitive reactions, along with non-steroidal anti-inflammatory drugs (NSAIDs), codeine and blood strain medicine, particularly ACE inhibitors.

Quick modifications in frame temperature because of warmth, bloodless or bodily activity.

Viral infections, along with the not bloodless or mononucleosis.

Allergies to different materials, like latex or detergents.

Hormonal issues, like modifications for your frame due

to pregnancy, menopause or thyroid sickness.

Autoimmune situations.

Chapter Three

What are the signs of hives (urticaria)?

Hives appearance distinctive relying at the man or woman and the situation. They can display up everywhere to your frame. Signs of hives consist of:

Red, raised welts or bumps at the pores and skin.

Blanching (the middle of the hive turns white whilst pressed).

Itchy pores and skin.

Swelling (angioedema).

What are the signs of swelling (angioedema)?

Signs of angioedema consist of:

- Puffy or swollen face, particularly the eyes and mouth.
- Digestive issues, along with stomach ache, diarrhea or nausea and vomiting.
- Swollen hands, toes or genitals.
- Swelling withinside the mouth, throat or airway

which could make it more difficult to breathe.

Foods: Many meals can cause reactions in human beings with sensitivities. Shellfish, fish, peanuts, tree nuts, soy, wheat, eggs and milk are common offenders.

Medications: Many medicines may also reason hives or angioedema. Common culprits consist of penicillin, aspirin, ibuprofen (Advil, Motrin IB, others), naproxen sodium (Aleve) and blood strain medicines.

Airborne allergens Pollen and different allergens which you breathe in can cause hives, every so often followed through top and decrease respiration tract signs.

Environmental factors: Examples consist of sunlight, vibration along with from the usage of a garden mower, warm showers or baths, strain at the pores and skin along with from tight garb or scratching, emotional stress, insect bites and workout.

Medical remedies or underlying situations: Hives and angioedema additionally every now and then arise in reaction to blood transfusions and infections with microorganism or viruses along with hepatitis and HIV.

Oftentimes, no particular reason may be identified, particularly withinside the case of continual hives.

Risk factors

Hives and angioedema are not. You can be at elevated hazard of hives and angioedema if you:

Have had hives or angioedema earlier than

Have had different hypersensitive reactions

Have an own circle of relative's records of hives, angioedema or hereditary angioedema

How are hives (urticaria) and swelling (angioedema) diagnosed?

Your physician can diagnose hives and swelling through searching at your pores and skin. Allergy assessments can assist become aware of what's triggering a reaction. Knowing the reason permit you to keep away from allergens, hives and swelling. Allergy assessments consist of:

Skin assessments: During this check, healthcare carriers check distinctive allergens to your pores and skin. If your pores and skin turn purple or swells, its manner you're allergic to that substance. This form of allergic reaction check is likewise referred to as a pores and skin prick or scratch check. Skin checking out isn't normally executed if hives are continual in nature.

Blood assessments: A blood check exams for particular antibodies for your blood. Your frame makes antibodies to combat off allergens. The system is a part of your immune machine — however in case your frame makes too many, it is able to reason hives and swelling.

What are the scientific functions of angioedema?

Symptoms and symptoms and symptoms of angioedema may also range barely among the distinctive forms of angioedema however in general, a few or all the following arise.

Marked swelling, generally across the eyes and mouth

Throat, tongue, hands, toes and/or genitals can be affected too

The pores and skin may also seem every day, i.e. no hives or some other rash

Swellings may also or won't be itchy

Swellings can be painful, smooth or burning

In excessive angioedema swelling of the throat and/or tongue may also make it hard to breath

Swelling of the liner of the intestinal tracts may also reason gastrointestinal ache and cramps

Some functions particular to the distinctive forms of angioedema are indexed below.

Angioedema kind Clinical functions

Acute allergic angioedema

Almost continually takes place with urticaria

Angioedema and urticaria each generally arise inside 1-2 hours of publicity to an allergen (exception is ACE inhibitor-brought on angioedema that generally takes place in the first week of remedy however can arise weeks to months later)

Reactions are generally self-restricting and subside inside 1-three days

Reactions will recur with repetitive exposures or publicity to cross-reactive materials

Chapter Four

Non-Allergic Drug Reaction

ACE inhibitor-brought on angioedema takes place without urticaria

Idiopathic/continual angioedema

Similar to acute allergic however angioedema maintains on routine and frequently no regarded reason is found

Hereditary angioedema

Patients frequently enjoy no signs till they attain puberty

Swellings can arise with none provocation or brought on through precipitating factors, along with nearby trauma, lively workout, emotional stress, alcohol, and hormonal factors (menstruation, pregnancy, estrogen)

Some sufferers may also get a transitory prodromal non-itchy rash, headache, visible disturbance or anxiety

Face, hands, arms, legs, genitals, digestive tract and airway can be affected; swellings unfold slowly and can closing for three-four days

Abdominal cramps, nausea, vomiting, trouble respiratory and infrequently urinary retention from swelling of inner tracts

Urticaria (wealing) does now no longer arise

The tendency to angioedema is much less said in adults

How are hives (urticaria) and swelling (angioedema) controlled or treated?

Most of the time, hives and swelling leave without remedy. Your healthcare company may endorse medicines and at-domestic care that will help you experience higher and decrease your probabilities of getting hives again. Treatments consist of:

Allergy medicines: Medicines referred to as antihistamines block histamine's outcomes to your frame. Antihistamines relieve itching from hives and save you hypersensitive reactions. Some antihistamines react fast, like diphenhydramine (Benadryl). Depending how excessive the hives are, your healthcare company may also endorse each day over-the-counter (OTC) or prescription allergic reaction medicines, like loratadine (Claritin). fexofenadine (Allegra), cetirizine (Zyrtec) or levocetirizine (Xyzal).

Allergy shots: For difficult-to-deal with continual hives, your healthcare company may also endorse a month-to-month injection of a drug referred to as omalizumab (Xolair). This medicine blocks the frame's allergic reaction antibody, immunoglobin E (IgE), from inflicting allergic reaction reactions. People with excessive hypersensitive reactions could make an excessive amount of IgE, main to issues like hives and asthma.

At-domestic remedies: To relieve hives, you may take a groovy or shower, put on loose-becoming garb and practice bloodless compresses. An OTC hydrocortisone cream, along with Cortizone, can relieve itching and swelling.

Epinephrine: Severe hypersensitive reactions and swelling can result in a life-threatening situation referred to as anaphylaxis. Symptoms consist of hives, swelling, shortness of breath, wheezing, vomiting and coffee blood strain. People experiencing anaphylaxis want an instantaneous epinephrine injection (EpiPen) to open a swollen airway.

Oral steroids: Corticosteroids, along with prednisone, can relieve hive signs that don't reply to antihistamines.

What are the headaches of hives (urticaria) and swelling (angioedema)?

Anyone who has an excessive hypersensitive reaction ought to have life-threatening swelling (angioedema) of the airlines —

your throat and lungs. This situation is called anaphylaxis. It can doubtlessly near off the airlines, ensuing in death.

Anaphylaxis is frequently prompted through an excessive hypersensitive reaction to a sure food, like peanuts and tree nuts, or a bee sting. People having anaphylaxis want an instantaneous shot of epinephrine, along with injectable epinephrine (EpiPen or AUVI-Q). Epinephrine opens airlines, increases blood strain and decreases hives and swelling. If epinephrine is used outdoor of the scientific setting, a ride to the ER is warranted, on the grounds that signs can go back if epinephrine wears off.

How can I save you hives (urticaria) and swelling (angioedema)?

Allergy assessments can assist your healthcare company discern out which materials bring about hives and swelling. Once you recognize your triggers, you may keep away from them. You may also need to:

Cut sure meals or beverages from your diet.

Reduce publicity to airborne allergens.

Switch to detergents and soaps without scents or dyes.

Avoid intense modifications in temperature.

Relax and take a wreck whilst you're harassed or overworked.

Wear loose-becoming, light-weight garb.

What is the prognosis (outlook) for human beings with hives and swelling?

For maximum human beings, hives don't reason critical issues. Children frequently outgrow hypersensitive reactions that reason hives.

For a few human beings, angioedema can reason anaphylaxis — excessive swelling of the airlines and lungs. People with this life-threatening situation have to deliver injectable epinephrine (EpiPen) to deal with excessive hypersensitive reactions.

The End